Reiki Secrets

A Guide to the Ancient Healing Art

By Randy Fetter, Reiki Master

Reiki Secrets

by Randy Fetter

Paperback ISBN 978-0-9966270-0-9

eBook ISBN 978-0-9966270-1-6

Printed in USA

Dedication

This book is dedicated to my wife, Beverly Fetter. Bev encouraged me to follow my passion and write this book. She has been the one person in this world who has supported me every step of the way and I am forever indebted.

I want to acknowledge my editors, Kristina Saewert and Jennifer Martin. Without their help and advice this book would not have been possible.

Table of Contents

Introduction

Reiki Secrets is written for anyone who wishes to learn about Reiki Healing Techniques, including self-healing. Reiki Secrets is also written to help assist current Reiki practitioners improve their Reiki technique.

Reiki is absolutely universal and anyone wishing to learn about Reiki will be successful after they receive a Reiki Attunement by a Reiki Master (Reiki Attunement will be discussed later in the book). Compared to other holistic healing modalities, Reiki is probably the easiest to learn. Reiki is both easy to learn and easy to practice.

My own journey into Reiki began when my daughter bought me a book on Reiki. My daughter, Jennifer, knew I was interested in Holistic Healing. My training in the past using Healing Techniques worked, but left me exhausted after giving someone a healing. Reiki was completely different. Reiki provided me with a method to use Universal Life Force Energy instead of using my own energy. Reiki invigorated me. When I gave a Reiki Healing to another person, they felt better and I had an abundance of energy. For me, Reiki was and still is magical.

Reiki is often times a calling. People become interested and find Reiki when they are ready. If you are reading this book, let me congratulate you on finding Reiki and learning about this amazing life healing journey. Through Reiki, you will be able to heal yourself, heal others, and become more relaxed. Reiki can help you to relieve stress, and leave you feeling much happier than you have been in a long time. Reiki truly is a gift to yourself and a gift lasts for the rest of your life!

Reiki is absolutely universal and anyone wishing to learn about Reiki will be successful after they receive a Reiki Attunement by a Reiki Master.

Reiki is a gift to yourself that lasts your entire Life!

My personal journey into Reiki started just over five years ago. Five years ago I was told by my doctor that I needed to have a knee replacement surgery in both of my knees. I was shown x-rays of my knees that confirmed both of my knees were bone-on-bone. I was on daily pain medication to manage the pain and receiving Cortisone shots every four months in order to function as normal as possible. As soon as I received my level 1 Reiki Attunement, I noticed a slow improvement in the pain. Each time I practiced on myself, I could feel the warmth passing from my hands into my knees, and the pain I previously felt would subside for a short period of time. After four months of practicing Reiki on myself, I was able to stop the Cortisone shots. After six months of practicing on myself, I was able to stop the pain medication all together. It has now been over five years and I still have not had either knee replaced, and am off all pain medications, and Cortisone shots. In fact, I recently completed a 5K race and am jogging. Do I believe in the power of Reiki Healing – ABSOLUTELY!

My intention in writing this book is to help you learn more about Reiki, and help you on your own personal journey. I hope this journey and your interest takes you to the point of learning Reiki. In this book I will share subtle Reiki Healing Secrets and techniques that will allow you to understand and practice Reiki easier, whether you are a beginner, or an experienced Reiki practitioner.

Beginners will benefit most by reading chapters one through seven, plus chapters nine, ten, and fourteen. Beginners are advised to wait on the additional chapters until they have received a Reiki Attunement.

Experienced Reiki practitioners will benefit most by reading chapters eight through fourteen. Chapter eleven will be especially beneficial.

Let this joyous healing journey begin…

Chapter One

What is Reiki?

Reiki pronounced Ray-Key is a "hands-on" natural healing where Universal Life Force Energy is channeled from the Reiki practitioner to the patient. Reiki is a holistic healing technique that is completely safe and non-intrusive. The Reiki practitioner either lays hands on or just above an area where energy is desired to be sent.

A Reiki practitioner is given Reiki Attunements, trained in the philosophy of Reiki, and taught how to properly give Reiki Healing Treatments. Reiki is very easy to learn, but like any discipline, Reiki requires practice, practice, and more practice to master.

Reiki Healing Treatments can be done anywhere, but are normally performed in an office or a home.

Treatments are performed fully clothed and normally done in a chair or on a message table.

Hands are placed gently on or just above an area to be treated. While doing treatments, Reiki practitioners will work with clients to make sure any areas that you are uncomfortable having touched are only treated with hands slightly above the area.

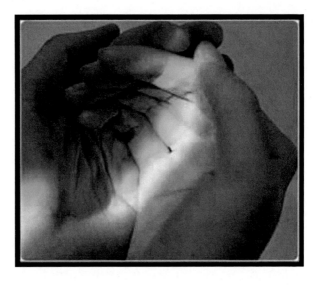

Reiki helps enable your body to naturally heal itself on a multitude of levels:

- Heal physical ailments, particularly the reduction of acute pain

- Brings the energy centers in both your body and spirit into balance

- Reducing stress

- Releasing emotional blockages

- Helps break bad or unwanted habits

- Brings the body, mind, and spirit into harmony

Receiving Reiki will usually feel either hot or cold energy coming from the practitioner's hands. I have had both of these sensations when I am receiving Reiki and both are equally nice, relaxing, and healing. Some people may feel nothing at all, yet will notice when the session is over that the sharp pains they felt before the treatment are no longer there. Reiki will treat a person on a physical, emotional, and spiritual level. For this reason, sometimes a person receiving Reiki will show emotion ranging from tears in their eyes to sobbing uncontrollably. Practitioners understand how powerful Reiki is and have each had the very same experiences as the patient.

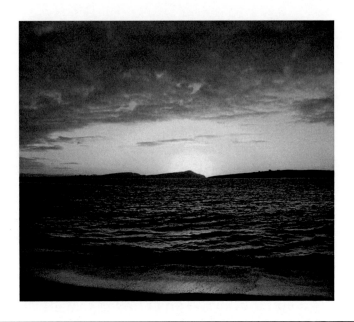

Reiki helps enable your body to naturally heal itself on a multitude of levels:

- **Heal physical ailments, particularly the reduction of acute pain**
- **Brings the energy centers in both your body and spirit into balance**
- **Reducing stress**
- **Releasing emotional blockages**
- **Helps break bad or unwanted habits**
- **Brings the body, mind, and spirit**

Reiki will work on anyone who wants to be treated, however, not at the expense of professional medical treatment or medication. Reiki will reinforce any treatment that is given and will help aid in the healing process. Those that do not wish a Reiki treatment, but receive one anyway normally do not receive any benefit. For this reason I do not suggest forcing anyone to receive a Reiki treatment unless they are open to the idea and actually want one.

So, if treatments only work for those that want one, does this mean it's all in our heads? Does this mean that Reiki is like the "sugar pill or placebo"? I have practiced Reiki on myself and I can personally attest that Reiki actually works and is not just a placebo. Reiki works on anyone wishing to receive a treatment. Since the energy transferring is slow moving, the drastic effects take time, while sharp pains may decrease almost immediately. For those that do not want a treatment, their energy might make the healing energy move much slower and delay or halt the long term affects. This is why treatments do not work on everyone.

An article in the Hartford Courant cites the results of studies done by University of Connecticut researchers on the effects that Reiki energy may or may not have on growth and proliferation at the cellular level. The researchers measured bone and tendon cells and tendon cells in the study. One set of cells was treated by a trained Reiki practitioner for 10 minutes twice a week. The second set was treated for the same length of time by a person that had not been trained in Reiki or Attuned. The third set of petri dishes was untouched as a control set. Several different biological markers for growth were analyzed, and in each test the cells treated with the Healing Touch of Reiki grew at a faster rate than the untreated cells. One test showed the growth rate was double compared to the untreated rate. The bone cells were able to absorb more calcium, which is essential for bone growth. The study essentially showed that Reiki energy can be linked to cellular growth and cellular healing.

> *The bone cells were able to absorb more calcium, which is essential for bone growth. The study essentially showed that Reiki energy can be linked to cellular growth and cellular healing.*

When students take a Reiki class to learn Reiki and receive an Attunement, the students often describe having upset stomach ranging from mild to a form of diarrhea. The queasiness may last up to twenty one days after the Attunement – almost without exception. My own experience was that I had loose stools for three days and an upset stomach for eighteen days. An Attunement is performed by a Reiki Master and is simply an infusion of energy. The energy is only transferred through the hands. Would this physical reaction happen to almost everyone if it were only imagined? I can assure you that Reiki is definitely for real.

The other advantage of Reiki is that once you have received a Reiki Attunement, you can treat yourself. This enables you to conduct your treatments at home, whenever it is convenient for you.

Chapter Two

Reiki History

No book on Reiki would be complete without discussing the history of Reiki. When learning about Reiki, I glossed over the history when I was in class. I wanted to jump ahead to the "good stuff". Eventually you will want to know who originally started Reiki and how the system of Reiki was learned by the founder.

Now that I am a Reiki Master, I understand the importance of having a basic knowledge of the history of Reiki. I have researched the history of Reiki and have attempted to share the basics without going into excessive detail.

Dr. Usui was born August 15, 1865 in the village of Taniaimura, which is in the Yamagata District, Cifi Perfecture of Kyoto, Japan. Dr. Mikao Usui is considered to be the person that started the traditional system of Reiki.

Dr. Mikao Usui held several different jobs during his life including; office worker, public servant, reporter, industrialist, politician's secretary, supervisor of convicts, and missionary. Mikao Usui was not always successful in business, even though he came from a wealthy family. Mikao studied in Europe, and China and his studies included medicine, psychology, religion, and divination. Dr. Mikao Usui had both a Christian and a Buddhist upbringing. He also studied Sanskrit, which is why we believe the sacred symbols are written in the manner they are. I will discuss the sacred symbols briefly later in this book.

Eventually, Dr. Mikao Usui became a Tendai Buddhist Priest. It is generally believed that Dr. Usui discovered the healing system of Reiki he taught based upon his life experiences and specifically the mystical experiences he encountered on Mount Kurama. Dr. Usui enrolled in a twenty one day training program called Isyu Guo, which took place on Mount Kurama. While the training is not shared with outsiders, it is generally accepted that the training would have involved extensive meditation, chanting, prayers, and fasting. After fasting for many days it is believed that Dr. Usui stood underneath a waterfall, allowing the water to continually strike the crown of his head while meditating. Dr. Usui believed that this opened up the crown chakra, greatly enhancing his ability to heal himself and others without depleting his own energy. In addition, Dr. Usui had a vision in which he saw several symbols on the last day of his twenty one day fast. The Reiki symbols he saw are taught to Reiki students at level 2, still to this day. (Those of us that honor the traditional system of Reiki do not share the symbols, except when teaching a formal class during the Reiki Level 2 and Reiki Master Courses). At the end of the 21 day fasting, it is rumored that Dr. Usui was excited to share his visions and started to run down the mountain. In his haste, he stubbed his toe on a rock and like any of us, bent down to rub out the pain. When he rubbed his toe he discovered a healing energy passing from his hands into his toes and the pain eased. As he continued the healing, his toe actually healed. Dr. Usui practiced his discovery on his family and through experimentation, refined his methods.

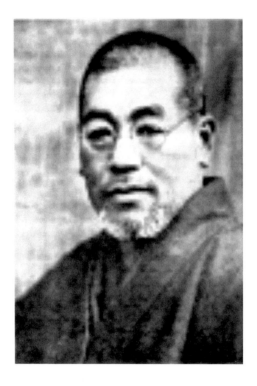

Dr. Usui then tried his healing system on the poor and indigent and found the Reiki system worked. However, Dr. Usui found that the healing worked even better when the receiver of the healing offered a token of payment. Dr. Mikao Usui started to teach the Reiki form of healing to a small group of students. The students were taught how to heal themselves and a small form of payment was offered in return. Dr. Usui moved to Tokyo in early 1922 and started a healing society named Usui Reiki Ryoho Gakkai. He taught classes and gave treatments. He kept detailed records and discovered which hand positions worked the best when treating patients.

At the end of the 21 day fasting, it is rumored that Dr. Usui was excited to share his visions and started to run down the mountain. In his haste, he stubbed his toe on a rock and like any of us, bent down to rub out the pain. When he rubbed his toe he discovered a healing energy passing from his hands into his toes and the pain eased. As he continued the healing, his toe actually healed.

Japan suffered a 7.9 earthquake in 1923 where the epicenter was 50 miles from Tokyo. Over 140,000 deaths were reported, with many more suffering injuries. Dr. Usui and his students started to give healings and as a result of this work his Reiki teachings grew in popularity. The demand for Dr. Usui's teaching became so great that by 1925, he had to open a new larger school in Nakano, which is outside of Tokyo. When Dr. Usui traveled, his senior students would take over his school and continue his teachings, while offering their services to walk in patients.

From my research, I have found that Reiki was passed on by Dr. Mikao Usui to Mr. Chujiro Hayashi. Mr. Hayashi was a commander in the Imperial Navy of Japan. Mr. Hayashi was appointed Reiki Grand Master and was responsible for leading all the other Reiki teachers by Dr. Mikao Usui.

Mr. Chujiro Hayashi taught and passed on the Reiki Grand Master to Hawayo H. Takata, who lived in Hawaii. Ms. Takata is credited with bringing Reiki to the West. Ms. Takata reportedly taught twenty two Masters before her death in 1980. Ms. Takata believed in charging a large fee to train others so that Reiki was valued, particularly in the West. Reiki is very easily learned and the system in essentially passed on by performing a Reiki Attunement, performed by a Reiki Master. So that Reiki was valued, she set up fees of $175 for level 1, $500 for level 2, and

$10,000 for those desiring to become a Reiki Master.

From here, Reiki branches off into several sects. It is important when finding a Reiki Master that you understand which form of Reiki they teach. All systems of Reiki work, but you will want to find a Reiki Master that resonates with you. I am biased toward the Usui system of Reiki since it is the purest form of Reiki.

Today fees vary greatly and are set by the Reiki Master teacher who teaches the course and performs the Reiki Attunement. There are now thousands of Reiki Masters worldwide and a simple search will likely result in several Reiki Masters within your own city. You will also want to compare the fees that are charged for the courses. Paying more does not necessarily equate to a better teacher or better course. What is important is that the teacher you find is interested in your development. You want to make sure the teacher is available to answer your questions. If possible, call the Reiki Master and talk for a few minutes to see if you have a connection that will be beneficial.

Chapter Three

Reiki Philosophy

The Reiki Philosophy is a very simple one as taught by Dr. Mikao Usui and involves five basic mantras. The five mantras are:

1. Just for today, I will not get angry

2. Just for today, I will not worry

3. Be thankful and grateful for the many blessings we have

4. Work hard today and do my best

5. Be kind to others

If you practice these five mantras every day, your own happiness will improve and your life will be filled with less stress, thus healthier.

Anger: Since we are all human, we are bound to get angry at times. The majority of the time when we look back on a situation, we do not understand why we had such anger at the time. Let your anger be brief and direct your behavior toward improving the situation. Anger is sometimes there to motivate us to do something and improve a situation

Worry: Worry never helps a situation. Worry is a natural human instinct. Instead of spending time worrying, take action on what you can improve and what is under your own control. What you cannot control let go and let the universe handle it. I know this is easier said than done, but with practice you will find that you will get better at it and in the process become happier yourself. Worry can cripple a person, or it can simply help a person focus on a situation that needs their attention.

Thankfulness and Gratuity: Be thankful for what you have. I will discuss this more in my chapter titled Reiki Secrets. There is truth that the universe works with the laws of attraction. You will find that when you appreciate what you do have; your life will begin to attract even more blessings than it did before. It is important to remember that there will always be folks that have it better than you, but there are also folks that have it much worse than you.

Hard Work: When you work hard and do the best you can, you will always be regarded highly by others. What is even more important is that you will be regarded highly by yourself. Dr. Usui was more than likely referring to meditation when he wrote this mantra; however, hard work at whatever you doing will always bring satisfaction and rewards.

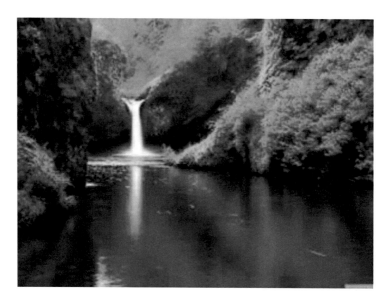

Kindness: Every religion in the world teaches the Golden Rule; treat others as you would like to have them treat you. Being kind to others will in turn result in others treating you well most of the time. This mantra does not mean to give everything to others; it means simply to be kind. You have the power to control your actions and responses and can politely turn down a request instead of cussing and getting angry. Those reactions seldom result in any improvement (except when you bang your thumb with a hammer by mistake).

Personally, I try to practice the five mantras every day. Many times I have failed. I have noticed by being aware of the mantras, over time I have improved. My life is a hundred times better today because of using Reiki. Reiki heals much more than the physical body. My emotions and spiritual health are vastly improved too. I still get angry, but not as often and the anger is less severe. I still worry at times, but not nearly as often. When I do worry, I try to let it motivate me to act in a positive manner.

The five mantras are:

1. Just for today, I will not get angry
2. Just for today, I will not worry
3. Be thankful and grateful for the many blessings we have
4. Work hard today and do my best
5. Be kind to others

Chapter Four

What Religion is Reiki?

Reiki is not a religion and works well with any religion in the world. Reiki does have some Buddhist and Taoist undertones, especially when learning the symbols. It should be pointed out that many believed Dr. Usui was a Christian and he certainly practiced Christianity for at least a brief period in time. Dr. Usui was also raised in a Buddhist Culture, and was a Buddhist priest. Healing will work regardless of which faith you possess.

> *Reiki is not a religion and works well with any religion in the world.*

At Reiki Share (where practitioners of Reiki practice on each other), usually every religion is present and Reiki works equally well with each of them. While Reiki is not a religion, it can cause a person to be more spiritual. Transferring universal life force energy and seeing the health improve in people shows each of us that there most certainly is something bigger than any single one of us. The universal life force energy is so plentiful that it will never run out or slow down. Seeing healing miracles happen with each treatment is bound to make individuals feel more spiritual.

Chapter Five

Reiki Degrees

In the most common Usui form of Reiki in the United States, there are three degrees of Reiki; Level I, Level II, and Level III/Reiki Master. There are several different branches of Reiki, which may offer more or fewer levels within their framework. Across all of these branches and levels however, the essential part of Reiki is to be able to heal yourself and others through energy. All Reiki is beneficial and no one branch is better than another.

Some branches offer more levels in an attempt to teach the finer details more thoroughly. Since I was personally trained in the most traditional form of Usui Reiki, I will only be discussing the three levels of Reiki.

Reiki is simple to learn because it is passed on from Reiki Master to Student through an Attunement, or initiation. An Attunement is a transmission of energy that essentially cleans the cobwebs out of your Chakras, thus enabling the Student to be able to channel Reiki "Universal Life Force Energy". Chakras are an energy field that is inside the body. Chakras spin in a circular motion and are located at specific points in the body. When Chakras move too slowly, ailments occur.

Once a person has received an Attunement they will be able to channel Reiki "Universal Life Force Energy" for the rest of their life. In my humble opinion, this is the very best gift you may give to yourself as your life will forever be changed in a positive manner.

You do need to be aware that once you receive a Reiki Attunement your life will change. Are you ready for this change? You thoughts will become clearer, your direction more focused, and you will learn a lot about yourself. Many people who embark on this journey will have relationship changes. As your health improves in both a physical and mental way, your dependency on others will diminish. This may sometimes affect the relationship.

> *Reiki is simple to learn because it is passed on from Reiki Master to Student through an Attunement, or initiation.*
>
> *You do need to be aware that once you receive a Reiki Attunement your life will change.*
>
> *As your health improves in both a physical and mental way, your dependency on others will diminish.*

I believe you are ready for this change or you would not be reading this book. Keep communication with those you love open during this process. People tend to grow together or grow apart. By keeping the communication open you improve the chances for growing together. Share your experiences, both the positive and the challenges.

Chapter Six

Level I Reiki

At Level I Reiki, the student is taught about:

1. The basics of Reiki

2. What Reiki does

3. A brief history of Reiki

4. The Chakras or energy centers

5. The placement of the hands during self-treatment

6. The student is given a Reiki I Attunement by the Reiki Master

At the completion of the course, the student will be able to perform Reiki on themselves as a result of having received an Attunement. The student will also be able to perform Reiki on loved ones and close friends. Normally students will not yet be ready to practice Reiki on people outside of their close network of family and friends.

> *At the completion of the course, the student will be able to perform Reiki on themselves as a result of having received an Attunement.*

The primary goal of Reiki I is to introduce the student to Reiki and allow the student to practice self-healing. Reiki is a natural healing method that helps heal all kinds of pain; physical, emotional, and spiritual. On physical pain, the results are normally fairly quick since these blockages respond well to treatment. Acute physical pain will be reduced almost immediately. The pain is reduced almost immediately, but may also return quickly at first. With additional treatments, the pain will be reduced for longer and longer periods of time. When physical pain does not respond well with Reiki, a medical doctor should be consulted. Although Reiki heals, sometimes a traditional form of medicine may be required.

The Wiley Online Library cites the Cochrane Library which states:

Touch therapies (Healing Touch, Therapeutic Touch and Reiki) for the treatment of pain relief for adults

Touch therapies (Healing Touch, Therapeutic Touch and Reiki) have been found to be useful in pain relief for adults and children. Pain is a global public health problem affecting the lives of large numbers of patients and their families. This review aims to evaluate the effectiveness of touch therapies for relieving pain, and determine the possible adverse effects of touch therapies. Although the lack of sufficient data means that the results are inconclusive, the evidence that does exist supports the use of touch therapies in pain relief. Studies involving more experienced practitioners tend to yield greater effects in pain reduction. It is also apparent that studies with greater effects are carried out by highly experienced Reiki practitioners. Further investigation should be conducted on whether or not a more experienced practitioner or a certain type of touch therapy provides better pain reduction. The claim that touch therapies reduce analgesic usage is substantially supported. The placebo effect has been also widely explored. No statistically significant placebo effect has yet been identified except through one study on children. The effect of touch therapies on pain relief in children requires further investigation. No adverse effect has yet been identified. This review suffers from a major limitation: the small number of studies and insufficient data. As a result of inadequate data, the effects of touch therapies cannot be clearly declared. This review shows that there is still a need for higher quality studies on the effectiveness of touch therapies in pain relief, especially studies on Healing Touch and Reiki. Future studies should make a concerted effort to systematically document side effects and report the experience of the practitioners to allow for the evaluation of the relationships between treatment effect and experience of practitioners. Future experiments should also follow the CONSORT statement when reporting in scientific journals, which helps to substantiate the reliability and validity of quality assessments.

———————

ClinicalTrials.gov is currently seeking to conduct studies to verify the effects of Reiki and states the following:

Complementary therapies such as Reiki are becoming popular. Reiki is a practice used for relaxation and pain management that involves physical touch and social contact with a trained, empathetic practitioner. Unlike many relaxation therapies, Reiki requires no participation by the patient, a feature that makes Reiki particularly attractive in the hospital setting, where patients are often extremely anxious, depressed, in pain, or sedated. Our primary research questions are to determine whether physiological changes are induced during a Reiki session and whether a Reiki session affects responses to a subsequent acute stressor. Secondary research questions include assessing which benefits result from placebo or unique abilities of "attuned" Reiki practitioners and assessing background characteristics of recipients that are associated with acceptance and responsiveness. Based on its use to reduce pain and anxiety, we will study potential mechanisms by which Reiki decreases activity of the sympathetic nervous system and other stress pathways. Comparison of the responses in a Reiki group with those in supine-control and sham groups will allow us to gain insights into mechanisms by which Reiki effects are mediated. Information obtained from the proposed studies will provide detailed information on physiological pathways affected by Reiki. Should Reiki decrease stress pathways or reduce physiological responses to stressful situations, it could be a useful adjunct to traditional medicine and have significant health and economic benefits.

ClinicalTrials.gov is currently seeking to conduct studies to verify the effects of Reiki and states the following: "Complementary therapies such as Reiki are becoming popular. Reiki is a practice used for relaxation and pain management that involves physical touch and social contact with a trained, empathetic practitioner. Unlike many relaxation therapies, Reiki requires no participation by the patient, a feature that makes Reiki particularly attractive in the hospital setting, where patients are often extremely anxious, depressed, in pain, or sedated."

Emotional pain will normally require a series of treatments over a period of time. Typically patients cry or sob during a treatment when dealing with emotional pain. Crying is simply a form of removing a blockage and enables the person to confront the emotional issue. Moving past painful issues does take time and cannot be accomplished in one visit or treatment. Treatments should be continued until they can finally move past the damage that had previously occurred. Spiritual advancement is an added benefit to receiving and practicing Reiki. Many students also report that over time they are able to sense other people's pain, even talking with those that are deceased, and developed a six sense.

Reiki does work miracles, but should never be contrary to medical or professional psychological treatment. It should be pointed out that Reiki does not take the place of traditional medical treatment, prescribed medical medication, or psychological advice. Reiki does however work well in conjunction with medical treatment. For this reason, Reiki is being added in more and more hospitals because of proven benefits. Studies show patients that have received Reiki are able to relax better, and heal faster. In the United States, Reiki is available at over one thousand hospitals as of this writing.

Once the student is trained on what Reiki does and the history of Reiki, the Reiki Master will perform an Attunement on the student. The Attunement is a sacred ceremony and the student is asked to sit quietly in a chair with their eyes closed while the Attunement is being performed. During the Attunement, the Reiki Master will use the sacred symbols and concentrate on cleaning out the Crown Chakra, as well as the area around the hands. At the end of this ceremony, the student will be able to practice Reiki for the rest of their life, as a result of the Attunement. The Attunement is the primary method of being able to allow others to perform Reiki. The student will normally feel a transformation of sorts occurring during and after the Reiki I Attunement. I saw a variety of lights during my own Reiki I Attunement even though my eyes were closed.

Following the Reiki I Attunement, the student is encouraged to drink plenty of clear liquids over the next twenty one days, as well as avoiding alcohol. Almost all students will experience an upset stomach for the next few weeks, as well as loose stools. The symptoms will subside after three weeks.

My own experience when I received a Reiki I Attunement was amazing. I saw a rainbow of lights flashing before me even though my eyes were closed. The internal feeling I had was calming like I was at peace and everything was right with the world. This furthered my belief that Reiki is magical. As I described earlier, I had the loose stools for a few days and an upset stomach for a few weeks after the Reiki I Attunement. I made sure to drink plenty of water. Even though I had an upset stomach, my energy was greatly improved. I felt happy and excited.

After the course, the student will be able to practice Reiki Self-Healing daily. After approximately four months, if the student desires, they will be ready for Reiki II.

Reiki I classes vary by instructor, but normally last about four hours. The Reiki Attunement portion of the class is done individually and normally takes approximately fifteen minutes.

Chapter Seven

Reiki II

Reiki II is a more advanced study of Reiki and enables the student to add more tools in their quest of natural healing. Reiki II starts with:

1. A review of what was learned in Reiki I

2. Meditation and breathing techniques

3. Learning the sacred Reiki II symbols

4. Learning distance healing

5. A Reiki II Attunement is performed by a Reiki Master on the student

6. An opportunity to practice Reiki on other students is normally part of the course

7. Students are taught about the etheric body and auras.

The review of what was learned in Reiki I is important because questions frequently arise about what was expected of Reiki and what actually occurred in the first training. Students are able to digest the information better hearing some of the information a second time. Truthfully, at first Reiki seems too good to be true. Many students are not quite sure if what they are experiencing is actually happening, or if they are imagining the whole experience. Reviewing what was learned and having others there to confirm is reassuring to many students.

Reiki II is a more advanced study of Reiki and enables the student to add more tools in their quest of natural healing Reiki II starts with:

1. **A review of what was learned in Reiki I**
2. **Meditation and breathing techniques**
3. **Learning the sacred Reiki II symbols**
4. **Learning distance healing**
5. **A Reiki II Attunement is performed by a Reiki Master on the student**

> **6. An opportunity to practice Reiki on other students is normally part of the course**
>
> **7. Students are taught about the etheric body and auras.**

There are three major sacred symbols taught in Reiki II and allow the student to improve their focus, improve grounding, improve healing, focus on harmony, improve mental focus, and to help perform long distance healing. The symbols are kept sacred and the students are asked not to share the symbols with those not yet trained in Reiki II. The symbols can be found, but do not appear to hold any power except to those that have received the Reiki II Attunement. This is probably because the sacred symbols are more of a method to focus intense energy, rather than really possessing any magical power.

In addition; the spirit words, or Mantras are taught in Reiki II that are associated with the sacred symbols. The sacred symbols and the Mantras improve the ability to increase Universal Life Force Energy toward the desired healing by creating a single focal point.

Distance Healing is taught to the student where they learn to use the sacred symbols to transmit healing energy to another that is at a distance. Distance Healing can be transmitted to a person in another room, State, or even Country. Distance Healing can also be done so that it arrives at a predetermined time in the future when energy is needed. As an example; a distance healing may be performed and arranged when a person is set to have an upcoming surgery. Distance Healing can also be sent in the past where it is particularly useful on healing past emotional trauma.

The student will again receive a Reiki Attunement. During the Reiki II Attunement, the student is again asked to keep their eyes closed. The Attunement performed by the Reiki Master is much quicker than the Reiki I Attunement and the student will find the effects are fairly mild as compared with the first Attunement. The student will normally experience a queasy stomach for a few days following the Attunement, but not the loose stools like the first time. The student is asked to drink plenty of water for the next twenty one days and to again refrain from alcohol for a few weeks.

Before the students are released from the class, they are given the opportunity to practice what they have learned in class on other students. In this manner, they both give and receive Reiki healing from others. They learn what it feels like to receive Reiki from others and are able to give feedback to those giving Reiki. This experience is invaluable as it enables each student to gain confidence in their own abilities as well as the abilities of others. The experience also reinforces that channeling Universal Life Force Energy is fairly easy once they have received the Attunements and that anyone is able to do so if they choose.

At the conclusion of the Reiki II class, the students are now ready to perform Reiki on others, including those that have never received Reiki. Most Reiki Masters will offer Reiki Share clinics where those that are trained in Reiki II may practice on other Reiki II practitioners. Confidence is gained and techniques are greatly improved at Reiki Share. Practitioners are reminded to respect the wishes of those receiving Reiki, including what areas of the body a person may not want touched. Practitioners are reminded that Reiki can also be given by placing hands slightly above an area being treated with the same positive healing results.

Once a person is Reiki II Attuned, this gift will last for the rest of their life. Many of those not wishing to teach or perform Reiki Attunements on others will choose to stay at the Reiki II level. For those that wish to continue on to the Reiki III/ Master Reiki level, they will need to practice regularly. Normally, a person is asked to wait at least two years before taking the Reiki III/ Master Reiki training.

> *Once a person is Reiki II Attuned, this gift will last for the rest of their life.*

The Reiki II course varies by teacher, but normally will be an eight-hour course. The Reiki II Attunement process is again done individually and normally takes about ten minutes.

My own experience when receiving a Reiki II Attunement was a disappointment. My Reiki I Attunement was exciting and magical, but the Reiki II Attunement was very subtle. I had expected the same magical experience as the first time. This time the Attunement was simply relaxing. Afterwards I noticed that the Reiki energy flowed easier. I also noticed more heat emitting from my hands when performing treatments. After talking with other people who have received the Reiki II Attunement, they also report the Attunement was more subtle. I had a mild upset stomach for a couple of weeks following the Reiki II Attunement, but much less severe than with the Reiki I Attunement.

Chapter Eight

Reiki III/ Master Reiki

Reiki III and Reiki Master are used interchangeably in the United States. Many people do not feel comfortable calling themselves a "Master", so they will refer to the Reiki III term. Becoming a Reiki Master enables you to:

1. Teach all levels of Reiki,

2. Pass Reiki Attunements onto all levels of Reiki students

3. Open a Reiki practice

4. Learn the Reiki Master symbol

5. Dedicate yourself to a life of Reiki

Becoming a Reiki Master should not be taken lightly and there is nothing wrong with deciding to stop at Reiki II. Becoming a Reiki Master comes with rewards and challenges. Passing Reiki onto others is a fantastic reward, particularly when you see the person develop and become happier and healthier. The challenges start with your inner self. There will be periods that you doubt your abilities and then whom do you turn to? After all, you are a Master. You tell yourself that you should know the answers. The truth is that no one ever is truly a Master. Reiki is a lifelong journey. There will always be new obstacles to overcome and difficulty for people to deal with. As a Master, you will be responsible for helping others on their journey. The inner strength of knowing the gift of healing and being able to pass this knowledge of Reiki onto others is exciting and exhilarating. I am reminded of the saying from several books and movies; most commonly known from the French philosopher Voltaire or Uncle Ben from the movie, Spider-Man "with great power comes great responsibility". Remember before embarking on this path that others will see you as a leader and a source of light. Make sure you are worthy of this trust.

> ## *Becoming a Reiki Master enables you to:*
>
> 1. **Teach all levels of Reiki,**
> 2. **Pass Reiki Attunements onto all levels of Reiki students**
> 3. **Open a Reiki practice**
> 4. **Learn the Reiki Master symbol**
> 5. **Dedicate yourself to a life of Reiki**

Of course, becoming a Reiki Master does not require you to teach or to do Attunements. Some people choose to take this step for their own personal journey. The Reiki III Attunement does enable even greater healing abilities. However, I believe that those that have taken the step to Reiki Master will be called at some point in their life to pass their knowledge onto others.

The Reiki Master course is normally two full days and involves:

1. Reviewing all of the material from Reiki I and Reiki II

2. Learning the Reiki Master symbol

3. Receiving the Reiki Master Attunement

4. Practice performing a Reiki Attunement on another person

5. Demonstrating a solid understanding of Reiki

Because of the quantity of material involved, certain Masters will require two weekends to conduct the course. In addition, normally a guide or manual is given to the students on how to teach Reiki to others at each level. At the conclusion of the course, although you will be qualified to teach, any Reiki Master will agree at least a year of practice will be needed before one is actually ready to begin to teach.

The Reiki Master Attunement is very subtle and the effects are mild as compared with the other Attunements. The universal life force energy that you will be able to channel will be greatly improved. This also means that the emotional baggage we each carry will be magnified for a period also. Since you will have to deal with the emotional baggage before you are ready to help others, at first it is recommended that you concentrate on yourself for a few months. Preparing yourself mentally for becoming a Reiki Master will also take time. Many Reiki Master Teachers will offer an Internship and it is highly recommended that newly trained Reiki Masters take advantage of the Internship.

My own experience when receiving the Reiki III/ Master Attunement was that this is the most subtle of all the Attunements. I did not experience an upset stomach afterward. The class was a great review of all the Reiki material. I learned some new techniques that have benefitted me. I did not feel ready to teach Reiki to others at the conclusion of the course even though I was now a Reiki Master.

At first, I went through a phase of self-doubt following the course. I did not feel any different than before taking the course. During the next few weeks a major change would occur. I noticed that the Life Force Energy now radiated from my hands even when I was not intentionally running Reiki. My healing powers were substantially improved. As part of my course, my Sensei offered to let me lead a couple of Reiki Share classes. Reiki Share classes are when Reiki practitioners practice on each other. The Reiki Share classes went well and I gained my confidence back.

As a Reiki Master my responsibility is to help others heal and learn Reiki. I do not have all the answers. I do have the ability to channel Universal Life Force Energy and that has been the greatest gift of all.

I am often asked; "What is so great about Reiki?"

My answer is that I am able to heal others and to heal myself. Reiki is truly magical. When I channel Universal Life Force Energy, not only am I healing another person or animal, I am also healing myself. The healing is a complete system; Reiki heals injuries, aches, pains, emotional pain, and heals the Spirit. What could be more magical than that?

> *I am often asked; "What is so great about Reiki?"*
>
> *My answer is that I am able to heal others and to heal myself. Reiki is truly magical.*

Chapter Nine

Meditation

Meditation is not required to practice Reiki, but knowing how to meditate greatly improves the flow of energy from the Reiki practitioner to the patient. Meditation is a method that allows you to quiet and cleanse your mind. Science has also proven through the use of scans, meditation activates other areas of the brain, improving functionality in a multitude of tasks. The following is an article from the Harvard Gazette dated January 21, 2011 by Sue McGreevy, MGH Communications:

Eight weeks to a better brain

Meditation study shows changes associated with awareness, stress

Participating in an eight-week mindfulness meditation program appears to make measurable changes in brain regions associated with memory, sense of self, empathy, and stress. In a study that will appear in the Jan. 30 issue of Psychiatry Research: Neuroimaging, a team led by Harvard-affiliated researchers at Massachusetts General Hospital (MGH) reported the results of their study, the first to document meditation-produced changes over time in the brain's gray matter."

"This study demonstrates that changes in brain structure may underlie some of these reported improvements and that people are not just feeling better because they are spending time relaxing."

"Although the practice of meditation is associated with a sense of peacefulness and physical relaxation, practitioners have long claimed that meditation also provides cognitive and psychological benefits that persist throughout the day," says study senior author Sara Lazar of the MGH Psychiatric Neuroimaging Research Program and a Harvard Medical School instructor in psychology. "This study demonstrates that changes in brain structure may underlie some of these reported improvements and that people are not just feeling better because they are spending time relaxing."

Previous studies from Lazar's group and others found structural differences between the brains of experienced meditation practitioners and individuals with no history of meditation, observing thickening of the cerebral cortex in areas associated with attention and emotional integration. But those investigations could not document that those differences were actually produced by meditation.

For the current study, magnetic resonance (MR) images were taken of the brain structure of 16 study participants two weeks before and after they took part in the eight-week Mindfulness-Based Stress Reduction (MBSR) Program at the University of Massachusetts Center for Mindfulness. In addition to weekly meetings that included practice of mindfulness meditation — which focuses on nonjudgmental awareness of sensations, feelings, and state of mind — participants received audio recordings for guided meditation practice and were asked to keep track of how much time they practiced each day. A set of MR brain images was also taken of a control group of nonmeditators over a similar time interval.

Meditation group participants reported spending an average of 27 minutes each day practicing mindfulness exercises, and their responses to a mindfulness questionnaire indicated significant improvements compared with pre-participation responses. The analysis of MR images, which focused on areas where meditation-associated differences were seen in earlier studies, found increased gray-matter density in the hippocampus, known to be important for learning and memory, and in structures associated with self-awareness, compassion, and introspection.

Participant-reported reductions in stress also were correlated with decreased gray-matter density in the amygdala, which is known to play an important role in anxiety and stress. Although no change was seen in a self-awareness-associated structure called the insula, which had been identified in earlier studies, the authors suggest that longer-term meditation practice might be needed to produce changes in that area. None of these changes were seen in the control group, indicating that they had not resulted merely from the passage of time.

"It is fascinating to see the brain's plasticity and that, by practicing meditation, we can play an active role in changing the brain and can increase our well-being and quality of life," says Britta Hölzel, first author of the paper and a research fellow at MGH and Giessen University in Germany. "Other studies in different patient populations have shown that meditation can make significant improvements in a variety of symptoms, and we are now investigating the underlying mechanisms in the brain that facilitate this change."

Amishi Jha, a University of Miami neuroscientist who investigates mindfulness-training's effects on individuals in high-stress situations, says, "These results shed light on the mechanisms of action of mindfulness-based training. They demonstrate that the first-person experience of stress can not only be reduced with an eight-week mindfulness training program but that this experiential change corresponds with structural changes in the amygdala, a finding that opens doors to many possibilities for further research on MBSR's potential to protect against stress-related disorders, such as post-traumatic stress disorder." Jha was not one of the study investigators.

James Carmody of the Center for Mindfulness at University of Massachusetts Medical School is one of the co-authors of the study, which was supported by the National, the British Broadcasting Company, and the Mind and Life Institute. For more information on the work of Lazar's team.

Simply being able to quiet the mind for brief periods helps to alleviate stress, lower blood pressure, and improve feelings of well-being.

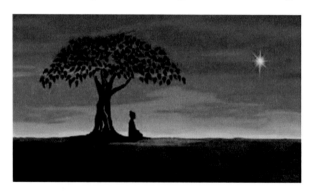

Some people have difficulty learning to meditate because they cannot quiet their mind. Meditation does take practice. No one is born with the knowledge of how to meditate. The difficulty you have when meditating for the first time will gradually improve. After a few short weeks, meditation will become easy and you will wonder why meditating was ever difficult.

Like all disciplines, the trick to being successful is starting slow. Here are some methods to help you get started:

Breathing: Only concentrate on your breathing; try not to think of anything else.

(In the beginning, your mind may wander. Just keep bringing your focus back and concentrate on this breathing exercise).

Breathing Exercise:

1. Find a comfortable place where you may sit in a relaxed state and not be interrupted for 15 minutes.

2. Relax your muscles and close your eyes.

3. Breathe in deeply to a count of 7

4. Hold your breath to a count of 7

5. Breathe out deeply to a count of 7

6. After doing this for 7 times, breathe normally for a few minutes, and then repeat

7. Continue this routine for 15 minutes.

8. If at any time you get dizzy, just breathe normally for 30 seconds then start back to the routine.

After you have tried the breathing exercise for several weeks, try sitting quietly thinking about nothing. You will not be able to do this at first, so take a couple of deep breaths. When you notice your mind starting to wander, focus on the thought without judging it. Take a mental note and notice if you see any particular pattern. It is important not to judge the thought as good or bad – it just is. Continue this process for 15 minutes each day. The truth is that none of us actually are successful at thinking of nothing. Meditation does allow us to quiet the mind, and then focus on a single thought.

After approximately six weeks, you are ready to practice a meditation.

Meditation Exercise:

1. Find a quiet place where you can sit relaxed and not be disturbed for the next 30 minutes.

2. Close your eyes.

3. Sit quietly focusing only on your natural breathing.

4. When you are ready, envision yourself surrounded by a white light. The white light completely surrounds you and is full of warmth.

5. Breathe in the white light, taking a slow gentle breath in, and then exhaling.

6. Imagine the white light filling your lungs, then your heart, and slowly filling your entire body.

7. Enjoy the warmth and serenity the white light is giving your body.

8. If a thought enters your mind, explore the one single thought. Where does the thought take you? If you determine the thought is

not desirable, imagine an outcome that is desirable for this thought.

9. Concentrate again on the white light and the warmth you are experiencing.

10. After 30 minutes, allow the white light to dissipate.

11. Before leaving this quiet place, be sure to appreciate what you just experienced.

Meditation takes practice, so try to make this a daily routine. This is the time you give yourself – you are worthy of this time. Enjoy this gift that you give yourself. Occasionally, a thought will focus that has brought you difficulty in the past. Try not to judge the thought, just simply examine what is being brought into your mind. This is perfectly normal and everyone goes through a few tough periods. Continue to practice meditating daily and you will quickly move past any difficult issues.

This is the time you give yourself – you are worthy of this time. Enjoy this gift that you give yourself.

Finally, remember none of us are perfect. Do not be harsh on yourself for mistakes or wrongs you have done in the past. Learn from the mistakes so that they are not repeated. Focus on being a better YOU.

Chapter Ten

Reiki Treatment and Chakras

This chapter is dedicated to the placement of hands while channeling Reiki Universal Life Force Energy. I recommend using the hand placements shown here first; then, feel free to experiment on your own. The hand placements are typically along the line of the seven major chakras. Chakras are energy centers in the body where the energy spins. A slow moving Chakra is generally perceived to be a blockage, which frequently results in pain or illness. A Chakra spinning too quickly also may bring pain, such as a headache. On the next couple of pages are a couple of pictures that illustrate the seven major Chakras.

> *The hand placements are typically along the line of the seven major chakras. Chakras are energy centers in the body where the energy spins.*

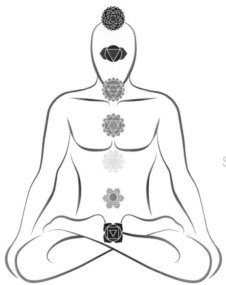

Crown Chakra

Third Eye Chakra

Throat Chakra

Heart Chakra

Solar Plexus Chakra

Sacral Chakra

Root Chakra

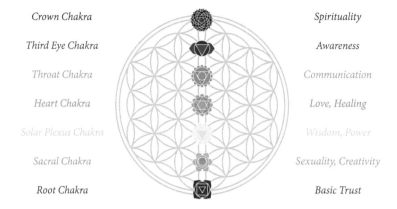

Crown Chakra		Spirituality
Third Eye Chakra		Awareness
Throat Chakra		Communication
Heart Chakra		Love, Healing
Solar Plexus Chakra		Wisdom, Power
Sacral Chakra		Sexuality, Creativity
Root Chakra		Basic Trust

Hand placements are used in Reiki treatments to help direct the Universal Life Force Energy. I recommend when placing hands that they are in a cupped position with fingers together. I also recommend that for the first few months, Reiki be done with your eyes closed. When giving Reiki to another person, only open your eyes when moving from one location of the body to the next. This brief period of open eyes allows you to respect the patient, as well as keeping you safe from any tripping hazards that may be present. Open eyes for the duration of a Reiki Healing Treatment should be reserved for experienced Reiki practitioners only.

The following are the hand placements that I recommend:

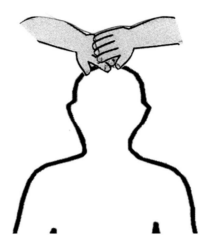

Position 1

Hands are placed directly on the Crown of the Head (Crown Chakra).

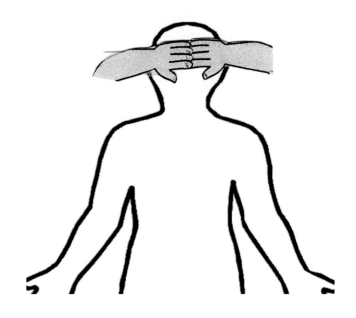

Position 2

Hands are placed above the eyes, where the third eye would be (Third Eye Chakra). Be careful to avoid any pressure on the eyes and the nose as this is uncomfortable for the patient.

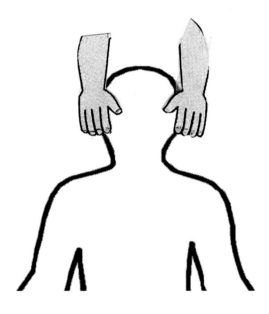

Position 3

Hands are placed over the ears in a cupped manner.

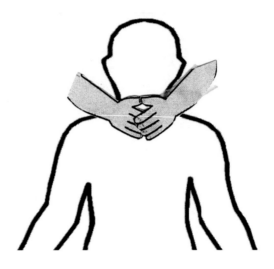

Position 4

Hands are placed gently on the throat (Throat Chakra). Be careful not to apply pressure as this will be uncomfortable for the patients.

When self-healing, it is best to cross your arms in a "X" manner; otherwise it is very difficult to do this on yourself.

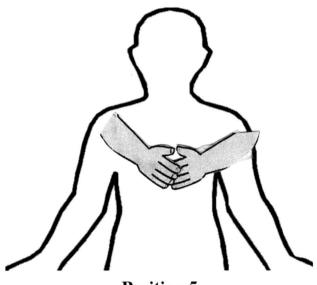

Position 5

Hands are placed in the center of the chest (Heart Chakra). When a female is being treated, to avoid the breast or private area, the hands should be placed above.

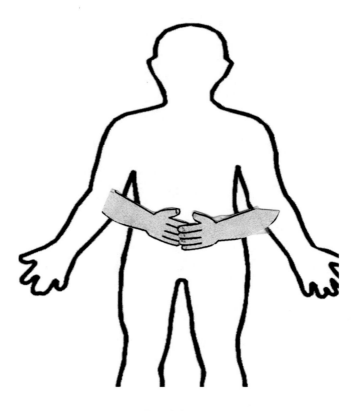

Position 6

Hands are placed just below the sternum (Solar Plexus Chakra).

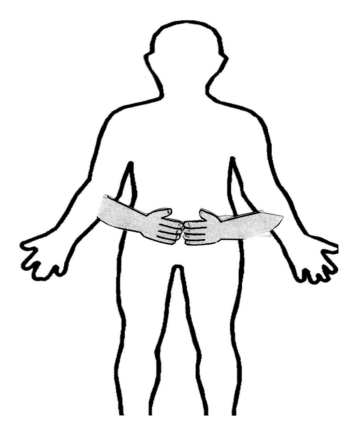

Position 7

Hands are placed just below the naval or belly button (Sacral Chakra).

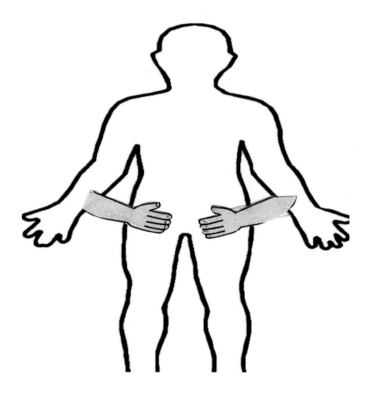

Position 8

Hands are placed above the Root Chakra. When doing a healing on others, hands should be "placed above" the root chakra area, since this area is considered private in all cultures. I have found that the area to the side where the pelvis is located works quite well when treating patients. It is important that the patient feels comfortable and safe when working in this area.

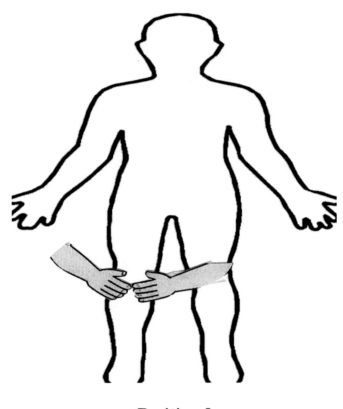

Position 9

Hands are placed on the knees. I normally do the
right knee first, then the left knee.

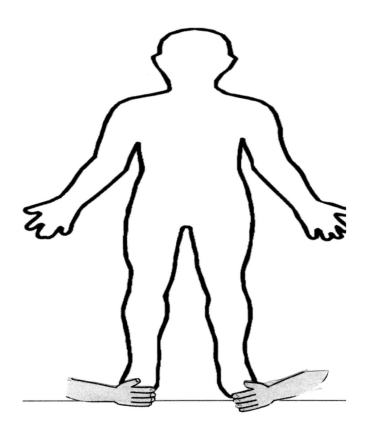

Position 10

Hands are placed on the bottoms of the feet. For self-healing this is virtually impossible.

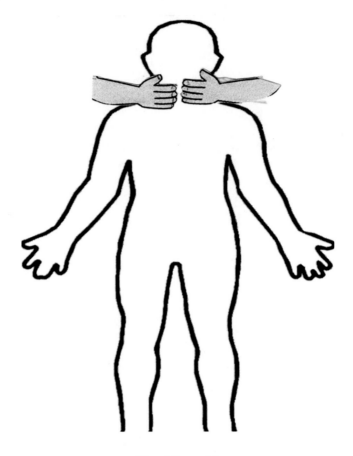

Position 11

Hands are placed on the back of the neck.

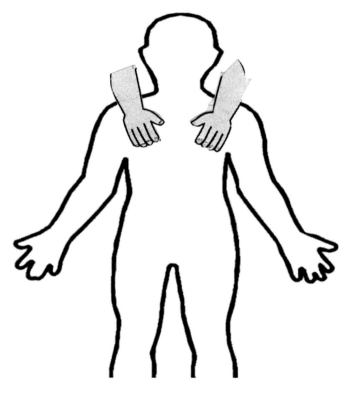

Position 12

Hands are placed along the shoulder blades.

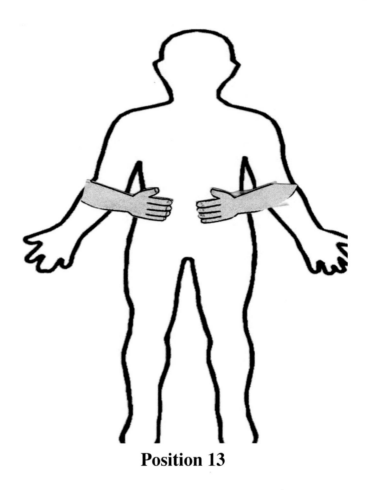

Position 13

Hands are placed on the small of the back.

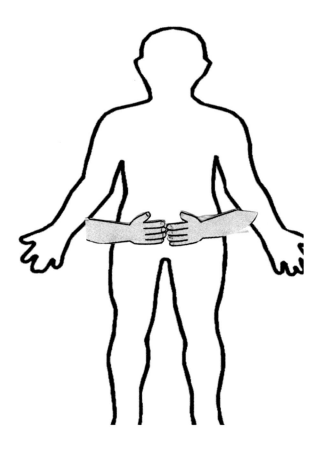

Position 14

Hands are placed near the tail bone. Be sure and ask permission first as this area is considered uncomfortable for patients in some cultures. If the patient considers this area uncomfortable, then place the hands above.

When finished treating these areas, always perform a "brushing away" of energy. This will start from the head and you will brush down toward the feet and side of the body to "brush" all unwanted energy away. Brushing is done slightly above the body of the patient. Be sure and ground yourself after giving treatments to others. The patient may be light headed, so assist the patient to a sitting position first and let them get their bearings before standing.

Chapter Eleven

Reiki Secrets

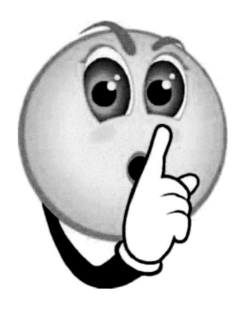

Secret 1:

Reiki is passed on by the use of a Reiki Attunement.

Reiki is very easy to use. Reiki is passed on from the Reiki Master through an Attunement to the student. The major secret of Reiki is that the Attunement is the one single act that empowers a person to be able to perform Reiki. There are a number of techniques that enable a person to perform Reiki better; however, the Attunement itself is what makes it possible to use Reiki. Once a person receives a Reiki Attunement they will be able to channel Reiki for the rest of their life. Reiki is a complete healing system.

Reiki healing is complete and pure, so another modality is not required. This does not mean the other healing modalities do not work, it simply means that a Reiki practitioner is not required to branch out for healing to work. Reiki treats all areas of the person; physical, mental, and spiritual. Although a Reiki practitioner may attempt to treat a specific illness, Reiki Universal Life Force Energy in channeled by the Reiki practitioner and goes where it is needed most. Remember, a Reiki practitioner is not using his or her own energy. They are channeling Universal Life Force Energy, which is the reason why Reiki practitioners are not drained at the end of a Reiki Healing Session, nor do they take on any of the illnesses they are treating.

Secret 2:

Protect the space before meeting with a client.

All of us carry an assortment of energies with us, so we want to make our space as neutral as possible. For this reason, before meeting with a client, clear and protect the space.

To protect and clear a space use the following exercise.

Protection of Space Exercise:

1. Sit calmly and clear your mind of any thoughts.

2. Envision white light entering the room.

3. Draw the white light into the whole room filling it with only white light.

4. Now see yourself inside a balloon.

5. Let only the white light inside the balloon and send all of the other energy outside the balloon.

6. Expand the balloon so that any unwanted energies are pushed outside of the room.

7. Ask that the balloon and the white light stay in the room until the session is over.

8. Protecting your space is widely underutilized. This technique also works when someone is invading your space, like tailgating you when driving. (Make sure to keep your eyes open if you are driving).

Secret 3:

Reiki works best if you are in a meditative state.

Before beginning Reiki, it is best to prepare by placing yourself into a meditative state. Being in a meditative state allows you to receive information intuitively and to direct the Reiki Universal Life Force Energy where it will heal the fastest. The truth about Reiki is, that even if you do not find the ideal place to start, Reiki will find its' way to the correct spot where it is needed most.

Hand position and knowing where to treat first simply supplies a more direct route so that healing may be done sooner.

Secret 4:

Reiki also enhances other special powers in the practitioner, so trust your intuition.

Your intuition will be improved as a result of practicing Reiki. Trust your intuition. As an example, if a client comes in and the client gives you a bad vibe, pay attention to your intuition and decline to treat this person. The truth is that there are a few bad people out there. Pay attention and do not compromise yourself. Never feel guilty for protecting yourself.

You may also find that you develop a six sense. This is perfectly normal and is actually quite common. I will get mental messages when I treat clients. If I believe the message I am receiving will benefit the client, I will ask the client if they would like me to share the message with them.

The client has the right to not hear a message I received mentally, so I never push the issue. Just be aware that developing a six sense is normal. Besides messages, one may also receive information regarding a patient another way.

When doing a healing, I also have the ability to see the color black in areas that need treating the most. While treating the black areas I sometimes receive a mental message that says the patient also needs to see a medical doctor. When receiving this message, I always advise the patient to have a medical doctor check out a specific area. I do not control whether the patient actually goes to a doctor, but my belief is that I would not have received the information if it was not meant to be shared with the patient.

Secret 5:

Channel Reiki Energy before beginning a session.

Use the following routine to channel Reiki energy before a Reiki Treatment Session begins:

1. Channel Reiki Universal Life Force Energy down through the Crown chakra.

2. Channel the energy down into the Third Eye chakra.

3. Continue to channel the energy down through the face.

4. Channel the energy down into the Throat chakra.

5. Continue to channel the Reiki energy down into the Heart chakra.

6. Channel the energy down into the Solar Plexus chakra.

7. Draw the energy down into the Sacral chakra.

8. Now draw the energy into the Root chakra.

9. Continue drawing the energy all the way down through the knees, and the feet.

10. Draw the energy back up through the back and down into the arms.

11. Finally draw the Reiki energy into the hands until it is flowing out of the palm of your hands.

Secret 6:

Make sure a person actually wants to receive Reiki before beginning a Reiki healing.

Always reaffirm that the person receiving Reiki actually "wants" to receive Reiki by asking them verbally out loud, "Would you like to receive a Reiki Healing".

Wait for the person to respond in the affirmative before proceeding.

In the case of distance healing, I always ask ahead of time if Reiki is desired, and then agree upon a time that the person receiving Reiki will be in a quiet area. Reiki II gives us a symbol that allows Reiki to be given over great distances and time. Distance healing can be given to another person that is physically in another location or country. Distance healing can also be sent to arrive at a specific time in the future, such as a surgery that is planned.

Reiki does not appear to work on anyone that does not wish to receive it. By affirming that the patient desires to receive Reiki, you can assume the healing works well. I am honoring the patient's wishes.

Secret 7:

Before starting Reiki, always ask that the Reiki be used for the person's highest and best good.

I normally affirm this statement out loud, "Please allow this Reiki to be used for (name of person) best and highest good". In this manner, I can be sure that I am not attracting any unwanted energies. By using this process, I also am affirming that my channel for Reiki Universal Life Force Energy is now open. I am asking the person's Spirit Guide to direct the Reiki Energy for the person's best and highest good.

Sometimes a person's best and highest good may be that their spirit needs to be healed rather than the injury they sought treatment for. I do not judge how the Reiki Energy is used. I simply trust that the energy will be directed where it is the most beneficial for my patient.

There are also times when a person may verbally express they want to be healed, but in reality they do not. This may be due to the person thriving on the attention they receive by being ill. Or it may be due to a karmic event, or this may even be this person's life destiny. Again, my goal is not to judge. I simply channel the Reiki and ask that the Reiki be directed for the person's highest good.

Secret 8:

Set the space with nurturing love to improve the Reiki treatment.

To improve the quality of the Reiki, a secret I use is to infuse a nurturing love into the space. I do this by silently asking that love fill the space. I do not start the session until I can feel and sense the nurturing love. Since there are many types of love, I specify that the love be a nurturing and healing love. Being a Reiki practitioner means that I carry a responsibility to make sure the environment is safe – safe for the client and safe for me. I always want to honor Reiki by ensuring that I never cross the line with the client. Some patients may transfer their feelings when they are being healed and start feeling a romantic love for their healer. It's important that one never allows the patient to be confused. I absolutely never pursue a relationship with a client. I do however; infuse the space by channeling a nurturing love mentally. This nurturing love improves the Reiki treatment significantly, plus as an added benefit; the clients do not seem to develop the undesired romantic love transference.

Secret 9:

Start by performing an intuitive scan of the client.

It is always best to perform an intuitive "scan" of
the person receiving Reiki. This is done by
placing the hands several inches above the person
and moving the hands slowly from the head
towards the toes. Areas that need to be treated will
actually "feel" different. Describing the different
feeling is difficult to place into words; however, I
can attest that the energy will feel substantially
different. The area that needs the treatment most
will feel different from the rest of the body.
Typically, the energy will dip where the person
needs the Reiki healing most. I will still cover all
of the areas mentioned in my chapter about hand
placements, but I will spend some extra time on
the areas where my intuitive scan showed me need
extra healing energy is needed.

At times this may mean that the session will go a
little longer than originally planned. I do not
charge extra when more time is needed, but I do
make sure the patient is okay with staying a little
longer, since they may have a tight schedule.

Secret 10:

The more you practice Reiki, the better you will become.

With experience also comes trust. The more often you do Reiki, the better your skills will become. You will get better at sensing where to direct Reiki and know when the Reiki is flowing well. Trust your own gifts as well. For instance; I have the ability to actually "see" where a person is having issues. In addition to the intuitive scan with the hands I perform a scan visually with my eyes closed. I am able to see the color black where the person is having a physical ailment. Honestly, at first I thought I was imagining this. With practice I learned what I saw was accurate. In this manner, Reiki gives each of us special gifts that we can use to help heal others. Each person has a unique gift. Be open to what your own gift is.

Secret 11:

Ask the client to take two deep breathes to improve the flow of Reiki.

When Reiki is not flowing well, a Reiki Secret I use it to ask the person receiving Reiki to take two deep breaths. Almost immediately following taking the two deep breaths, the Reiki will begin to flow deeply. I have often tried to reason why this method works, but with little success. All I know is that the two deep-breath technique works universally almost all of the time.

This simple technique is like working magic. Make sure you remember this useful tool when treating others, as this simple technique is the best secret I can share with you.

Secret 12:

For a blockage, use the Violet Breath technique.

When an area of the body has a dip in energy that is not responding well to the typical Reiki treatment, I have found that you can physically pull the negative energy out. To do this, you simply turn your hand away from the person and gently pull the energy out of the body. *Caution: be sure to direct this negative energy away from the person.* Once the negative energy is removed, you must send an infusion of positive energy to the area or it will reabsorb the negative energy again.

An infusion of positive energy is done by what is termed the "Violet Breath" by the practitioner. In order to use the Violet Breath, the practitioner must contact the Hui Yin point, (near the root chakra), plus place their own tongue against the roof of their own mouth. The practitioner then draws in white clearing light through their crown chakra, flowing all the way down through each chakra to the root chakra. The practitioner then envisions a violet breath and blows this violet breath into the area that needs to be infused with positive energy. I only use this technique when I specially need it.

As a suggestion, a gentle warning to the person receiving this may be useful so that they are not startled when you start to blow on them. At the end of the session, be sure to ground yourself so that you do not absorb any unwanted energies.

Secret 13:

Use an angled technique when a Reiki treatment feels off.

Sometimes you will feel the Reiki flowing, but something will feel "off". It will feel like you are forcing the Reiki into the person rather than having it flow easily. After asking the client to take two deep breathes, if I am still having difficulty, I will use an angled technique. I have found that by placing the hands on the side of at angles that the Reiki energy will flow better. It's almost like the person is tilted. Their chakras are spinning, they have plenty of energy, but the energy is not balanced. For instance; by placing one hand on the left side by the shoulder and the other hand by their ribs, Reiki energy will flow again naturally. I will keep doing this method by going down the body at angles. At the end of the session, everything will be back in balance.

Secret 14:

Scan a client's aura in addition to their body.

When doing a virtual scan of the patient's body, remember to scan their aura also. The aura is an energy field that surrounds the body. Some people are able to see a person's aura, but most of us feel a person's aura similar to a magnetic field. Where energy needs be added, there will be a dip in the person's aura. When a person's aura is too excessive, there will be a very sharp spike in the energy. To add energy to the aura, simply run Reiki with hands above the area. Where energy needs to be siphoned off, simply turn your hands away from the person and allow the energy to dissipate. Near the end of the session, do a smoothing of the aura field by moving your hands (hands above the body) in a circular motion starting at the head and continuing on toward the toes.

Secret 15:

Grounding after a Reiki session is helpful.

At the end of the Reiki Session, always ground the patient and yourself. By grounding, you are allowing any residual energy to be gently absorbed back into the Earth. Many clients will feel light headed following a Reiki treatment, so doing grounding exercise will help them return to normal. Grounding will also ensure that you do not take away any negative energy that the client brought with them. Grounding can be done by doing the following exercise:

Grounding Exercise:

1. Standing or sitting with the soles of your feet on the floor (ground), imagine yourself as a tree.

2. Grow roots from the bottom of your feet into the earth below.

3. Continue to place the roots deeper and deeper.

4. In order to check that you are grounded, slowly sway back and forth. You should feel completely secure.

5. If you are not secure, then grow the roots even deeper until you do feel firm.

6. Allow any excess or unwanted energy to flow into the earth.

7. When you are ready, allow the deep roots to drop away until you are normal again.

Secret 16:

Be appreciative.

Be appreciative for the Reiki healing. Be appreciative that another person has allowed you to perform a Reiki healing on them. Be appreciative for all that you have. I find that by being thankful at the end of a session that the Reiki Treatment is greatly improved. I typically do this silently unless I am in a group setting.

Be thankful in life too. We are constantly bombarded with commercial ads telling us what we should want and need. Too often we get swept up on what we do not have and the negatives in life. It is important to remind ourselves and others of all that we have. Practice a little thankfulness each day and your life will improve greatly. You will also attract positive energy into your sphere. A little thankfulness works wonders.

Secret 17:

Reiki is a complete healing system.

Because Reiki is easy to learn compared to other modalities of healing, many people practicing Reiki will also branch out to some other modalities. One of the most common is crystal healing. It is even rumored, but not confirmed that Dr. Mikao Usui used crystals in his early treatment of patients. This involves using specific crystals to aid in the healing treatments and an in depth understanding of which crystal is needed for which ailment. Others may use shamanism, angel healing, massage, and many others. No one method of healing is better than another. They all work to differing degrees or they would not be shared. Use what works best for you and listen to your calling.

Just understand the Reiki is a complete healing system and another modality is not required.

Secret 18:

Sometimes a person may have an unwanted evil energy that needs to be removed completely.

To rid an evil energy, the following exercise should be used.

Rid an Evil Energy Exercise:

1. Place yourself in a meditative state

2. Protect your space by surrounding yourself with white light.

3. Envision yourself inside a protective balloon filled with white light.

4. When you are ready, envision a black iron box.

5. Find the evil energy and place the evil energy inside the black iron box.

6. Placing the evil energy in the box may be difficult, so repeated tries may be required.

7. Once the evil energy is inside the black box, seal the lid shut.

8. Send the entire sealed black box to the other side of the universe where it will not ever return.

9. See yourself again completely covered in white light.

10. Come out of the meditative state.

11. Ground yourself.

Secret 19:

Sometimes there are people that are like energy vampires.

Energy vampire is a name coined for people that suck the energy out of you. After speaking to an energy vampire you feel drained. Frequently, these people are family members or loved ones. They often are people who have abused you in the past, either physically or mentally. You feel drained for months or even years after talking with them, yet you cannot stop thinking about them. The following exercise I call Cutting the Cord will help.

Cutting the Cord Exercise:

1. Put yourself in a meditative state.

2. See the person that is the energy vampire.

3. Look more carefully and you will see a cord or cords that are connecting you to them.

4. Now see a pair of scissors or shears.

5. Take the scissors and cut the cord.

6. Continue cutting the cord every few inches until no cords are attached to either one of you.

7. Be thankful that the cords are now cut and this person no longer affects you.

8. Come out of the meditative state.

9. Ground yourself.

Note: Be prepared to repeat this exercise every few days for the next few months. Energy vampires tend to grow cords back to those same people, so the cords will need to be cut in the future too.

Chapter Twelve

Treating Animals with Reiki

Animals can be successfully treated with Reiki. Since animals are more sensitive than humans, normally the Reiki will need to be with hands not touching the animal. You will need to intuitively ask the animal if they desire to be treated. If your intuition comes back with a yes, they want to be treated, and then begin to channel Reiki.

I normally will run Reiki and then show my hands to the animal. If they want to be treated they will move as close as they are comfortable toward my hands. If the animal keeps its distance, respect their space and simply run Reiki. The energy will go where it is most needed.

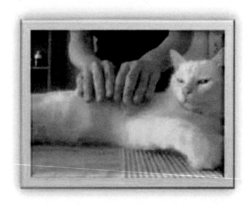

In rare instances, an animal will come all the way up to you when you are running Reiki and enjoy being touched for short periods of time. When the animal has had enough Reiki, they will leave of their own accord.

Please allow the animal to slowly get their distance. I have also found that dogs will thank you afterward by licking your hands gently when they have had enough healing. My own experience has only been on dogs and cats, but other animals may receive a Reiki Healings also.

Other Reiki Masters have shared with me they have performed Reiki on cows, horses, and even wild animals. Wild animals are always healed at a distance. Typically, even cows and horses should receive a Reiki Healing from a distance since they may be easily startled.

Chapter Thirteen

Treating Near Death Patients

As humans, we all have an expiration date—a date upon which our bodies will expire. Reiki heals patients universally; however, eventually we will all experience an end to our physical life on Earth. Treating patients that are near the end of their life also brings rewards. Reiki does not necessarily extend life, but Reiki does heal, relax, and alleviate the severity of pain.

As a Reiki Master, I am aware that I am only a channel for Reiki. My goal is to assist others by passing on Reiki Universal Life Force Energy and allowing others to experience the benefits of this miraculous gift. I do not judge since I do not possess all the answers. I cannot tell a patient when their time is over. What I can do is to offer a Reiki healing and witness the patient relaxing, enjoying a decrease in the severity of their physical and emotional pain, and being more at peace.

After experiencing a Reiki healing, the patient may pass away. Many times this is because the person has been holding on due to the emotional pain the patient can see their family experiencing. Many families will share that their loved ones crossed over after their family verbally expressed to the dying patient that it is okay to "let go". A Reiki healing may provide a similar experience, since the person will be at peace.

My beliefs are that Reiki has helped this person and that this is a part of life. The person has simply moved on. Remember, I stated earlier that Reiki is not a religion, but Reiki will make us more spiritual. You would not be able to channel Universal Life Force Energy if life simply failed once the physical body died. Reiki has proven to me that there is so much more to life and how we all affect each other.

Chapter Fourteen

Congratulations

By reading this book you have acknowledged that you are drawn to Reiki. Now is the time to act and answer this calling. If you are a beginner, find a respectable Reiki Master in your area and learn as much about Reiki as you can. There is a Reiki Master in almost every community, so you should not have to look far. A simple search should yield several excellent choices.

If you are an experienced Reiki practitioner, I hope that I have helped make your journey even more rewarding. I hope you found some new tools in the Reiki Secrets chapter that will assist you in your practice.

Remember, Reiki is a natural holistic method of healing. Reiki practitioners are able to channel Reiki, as Universal Life Force Energy using a simple hands-on healing technique. Reiki allows a person to give a hands-on holistic healing energy to another person without depleting their own energy or taking on any of the patient's ailments.

Reiki is a complete healing system. Reiki heals aches, pains, mental issues such as anxiety, emotional pain, and even spiritual healing.

Once a person has received a Reiki Attunement, they will be able to channel Reiki for the rest of their lives.

Meditation is a useful tool to aid in the channeling of Reiki, but is not a requirement. Practicing Reiki on a daily basis will also help you develop your intuition and many other gifts. Reiki is not a religion, but does amplify a person's spiritual journey. Reiki practitioners come from every single religion in the world and do not find any conflict with their religion while practicing Reiki.

The world needs more healers and I welcome you enthusiastically to the world of Reiki. Congratulations on improving your own life, and the lives of others!

Glossary

Attunement: A special initiation given at Reiki Level I, Reiki Level II, and Reiki Level III that opens a channel for the Reiki Healing energies to move through the Chakras and out through the hands.

Aura: A field of energy that surrounds the body of every living organism. Auras can be seen by some people. Most Reiki practitioners can feel or sense the aura similar to a magnetic field. Auras can be seen in Kirlian photography.

Chakra: An energy field that is inside the body and spins in a circular motion. When Chakras move too slowly, ailments occur.

Channel: A pathway that allows the energy to flow. In Reiki the practitioner does not use their own energy. Instead the Reiki practitioner channels universal life force energy for the purpose of healing.

Distant Healing: This method allows a Reiki practitioner to send Reiki healing energy to another person that is in another room, State, or Country. Distant healing may also be done in advance so that the energy arrives at a predetermined time in the future.

Life Force Energy: The energy that is vital for life to thrive.

Mantra: Words and sounds set off vibrational energy. Mantras are used in meditation or to add power to Reiki Healing Energy

Meditation: Meditation is a method that allows you to quiet and cleanse your mind. Typically the goal of meditation is to reach a state of "not thinking", to simply just be.

Mental Healing: The healing of the mind and emotions.

Sacrum: The bone plate above the cleft of the buttocks

Symbols: A symbol is a drawing. In Usui Reiki the symbols are considered sacred and are not shared until a person is Reiki II Attuned or above. The symbols allow a practitioner to improve their concentration and boost Reiki energy.

Universal Life Force Energy: The energy that is channeled in Reiki. Universal Life Force Energy is abundant in nature and can be channeled by any person that is Reiki Attuned.

Made in the USA
Middletown, DE
23 August 2015